Breastfeeding

ABC's

First paperback edition May 2024

Edited by Jillian Bray
Illustrations by Penny Weber
Book design by Veronica Scott

ISBN 13: 979-8-9906659-0-3 (hardcover)
ISBN 13: 979-8-9906659-1-0 (paperback)

The Breast Start LLC

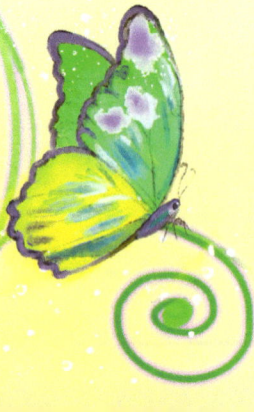

Breastfeeding ABC's

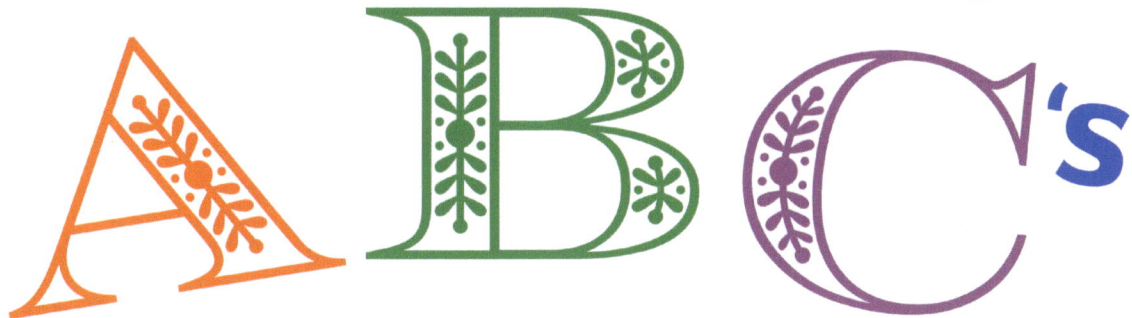

"The days are long,
but the years are short."
—*Gretchen Rubin*

Christsenio Dean RN, IBCLC
art by Penny Weber

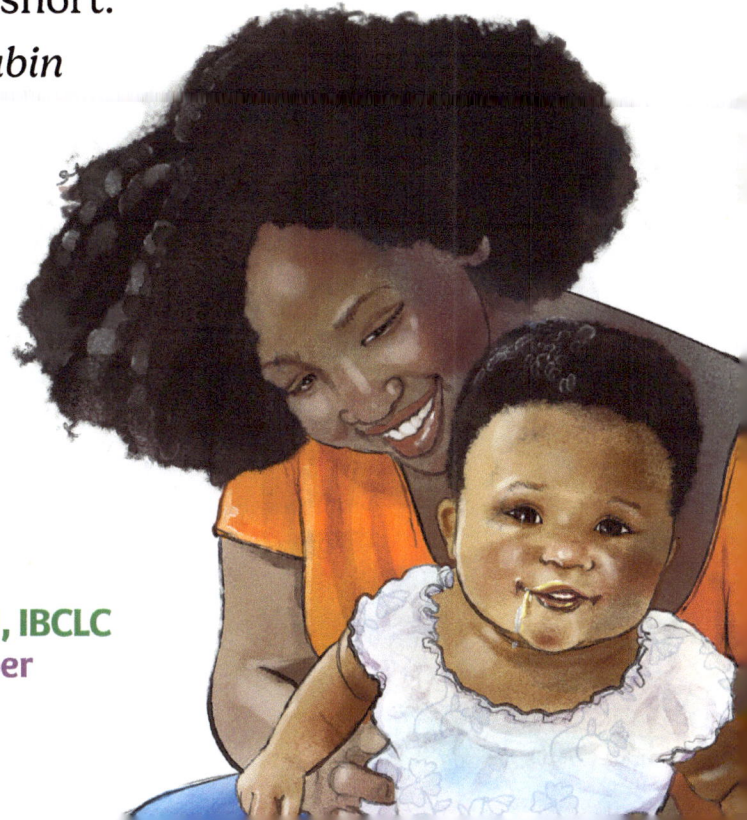

A

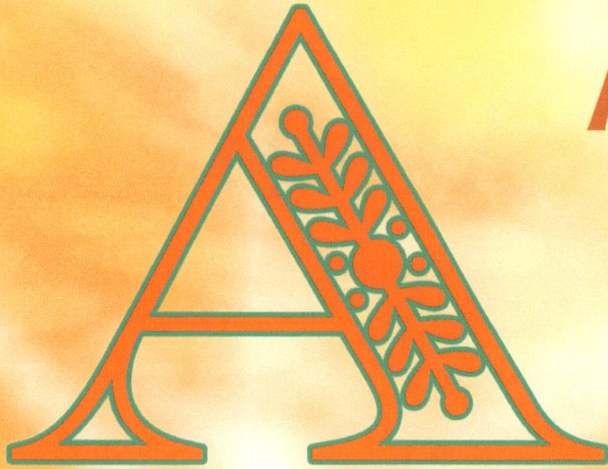

Attachment
Allergies
Available

Breastfeeding provides baby with **attachment**, or bonding, to mother. Breastfeeding can reduce **allergies** in the breastfed baby. Breast milk is readily **available**.

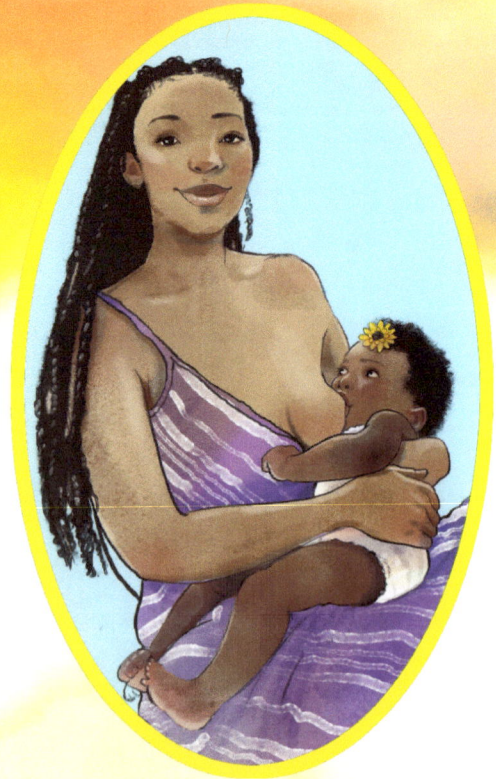

B

Breasts
Breast milk
Bond
Baby

Breasts make breast milk.
Breastfeeding creates a
unique bond between
mom and baby.

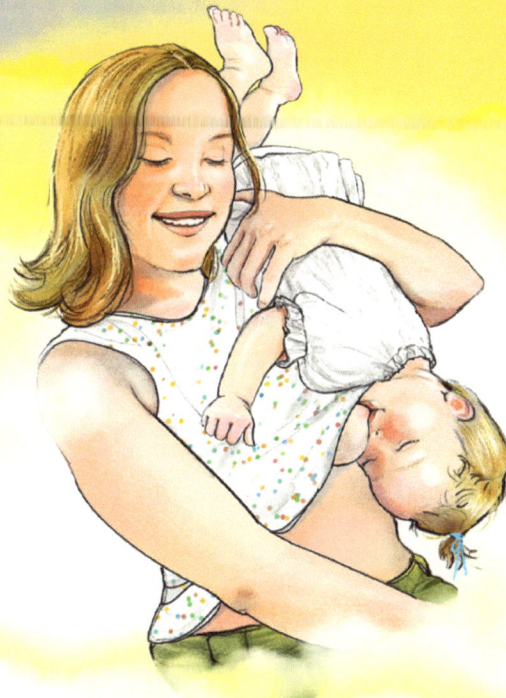

C

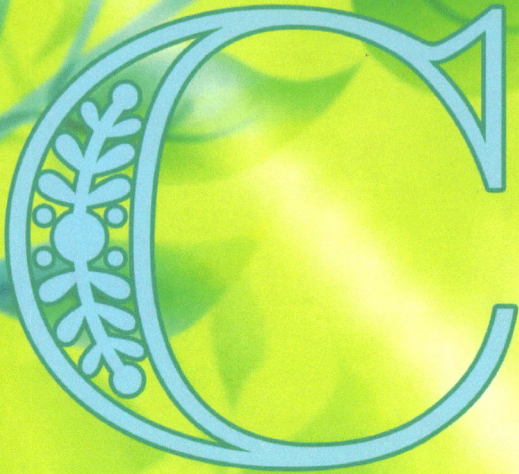

Calming Comfort Cuddles

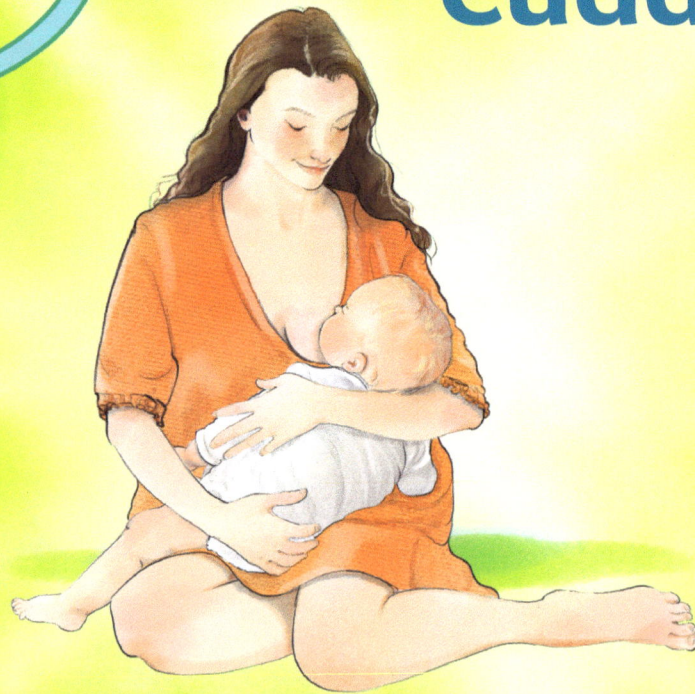

Breastfeeding is not only a source of nutrition but can also calm a crying, hurt baby. It provides comfort. Breastfeeding involves close contact and cuddles.

D

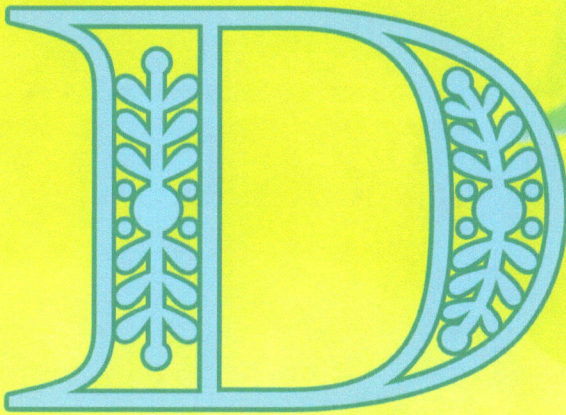

Drink
Dyad
Digestible

Breast milk is a **drink** for a thirsty baby.

A breastfeeding mother and her baby are called a **dyad**.

Breast milk is easily **digestible** by baby's body.

E

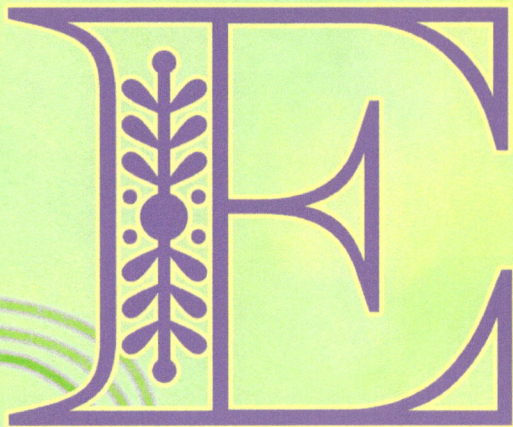

Empowering
Express
Eat

Breastfeeding is empowering. Many breastfeeding mothers are amazed by what their bodies can do. Milk comes, or is expressed, from breasts. Babies eat from the breasts.

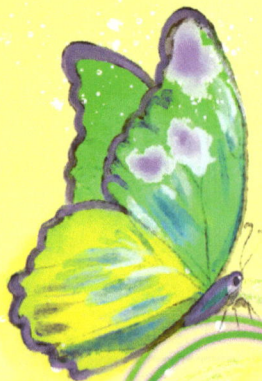

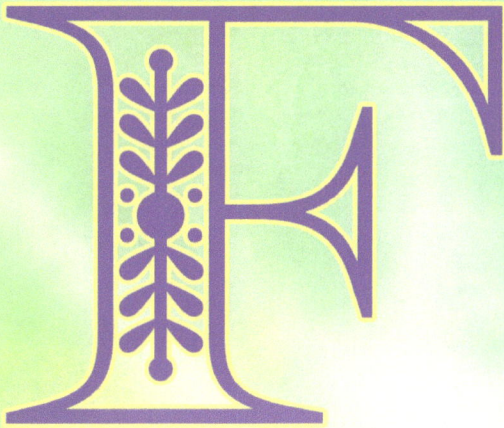

F

Food
Freeze

Breast milk is a food source.
Breast milk can be placed in the
freezer and stored for later use.

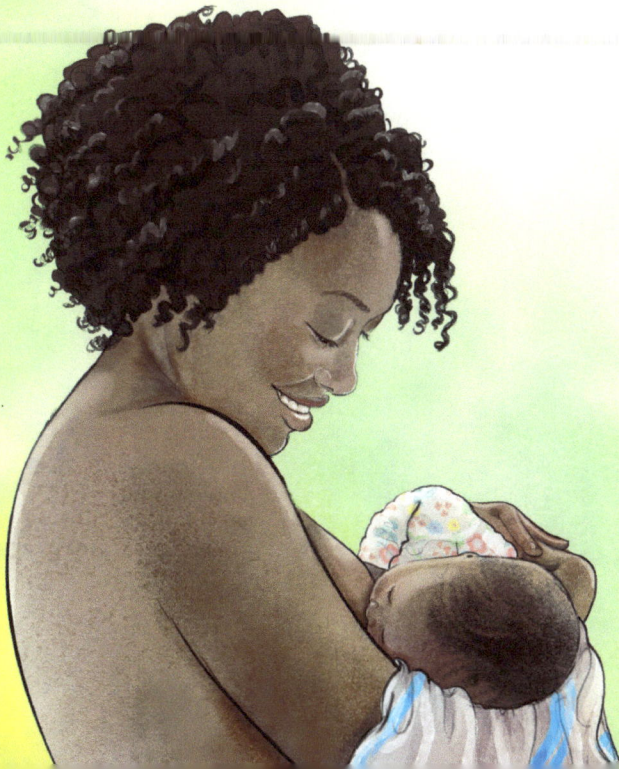

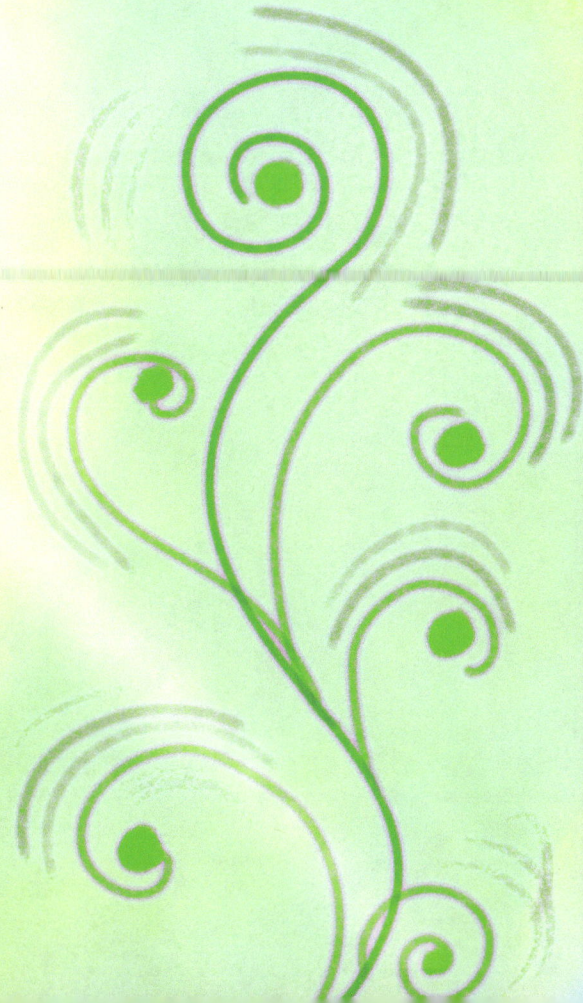

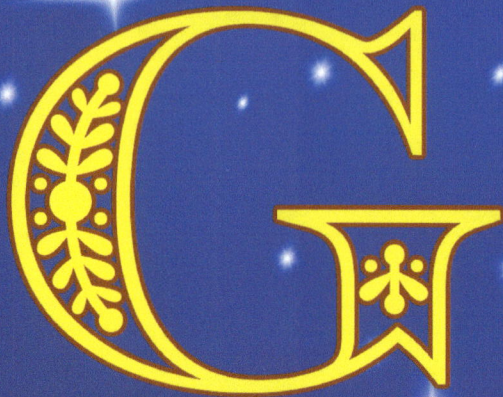

G

Gut
Goal

Breast milk is important for **gut** health. It provides healthy bacteria. Many breastfeeding moms set a goal for how long they wish to breastfeed. Whether the **goal** achieved is three months, six months, one year, or two years, it's a celebration and something to be proud of.

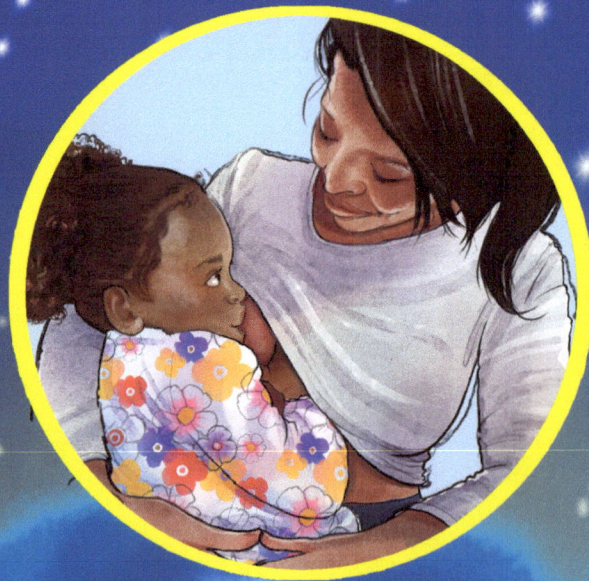

Hands
Healthy
Hungry

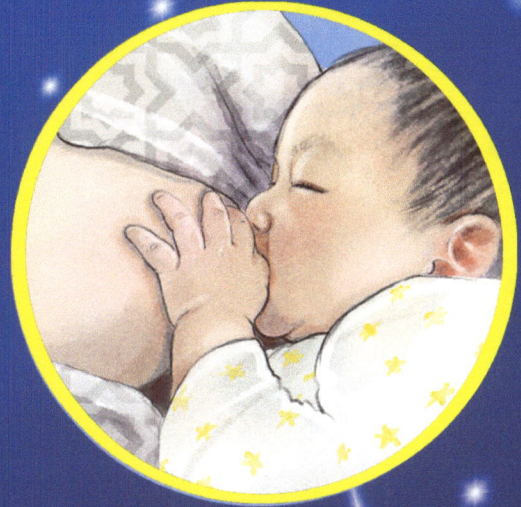

Babies use their hands while feeding, holding the breasts or twiddling the nipple. Breastfeeding is healthy for mom and baby. Babies eat when hungry.

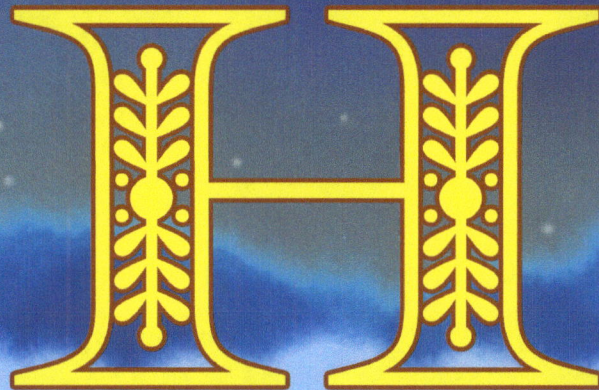

H

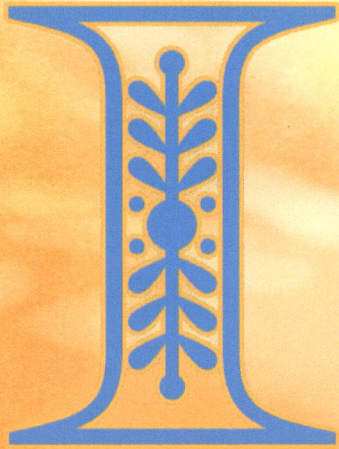

Immunity
Illness

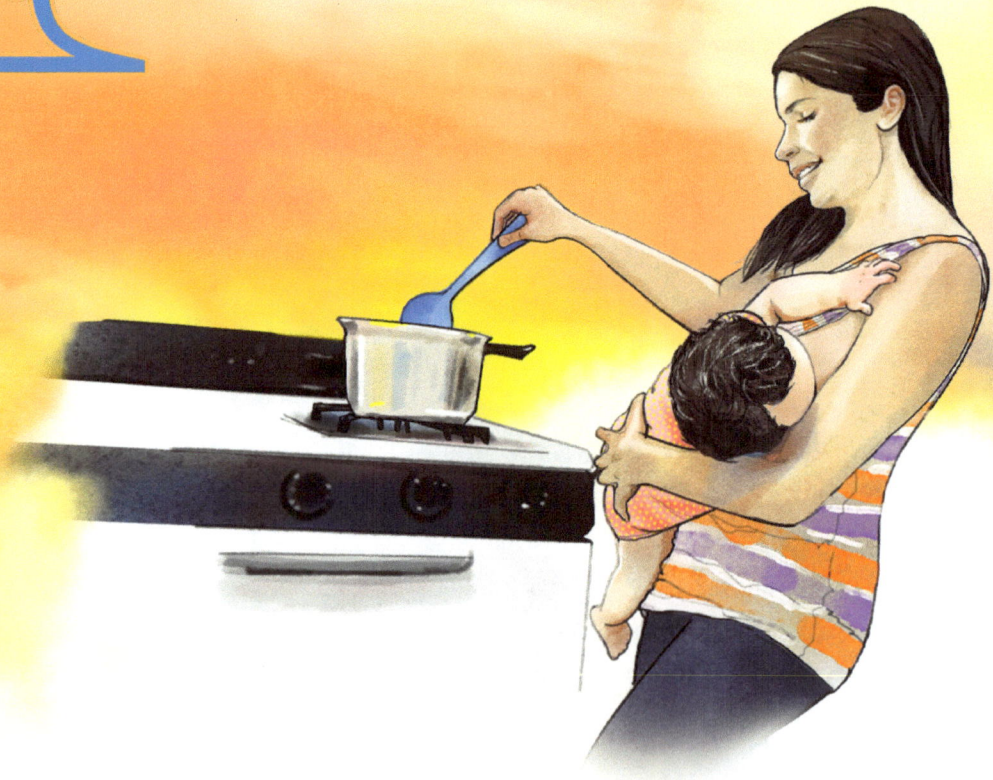

Breast milk provides baby with immunity, or protection against infection. It can reduce illness.

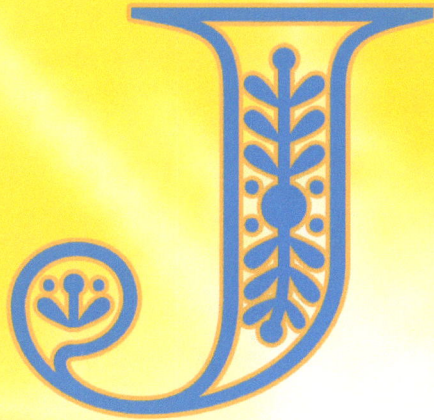

J Journey

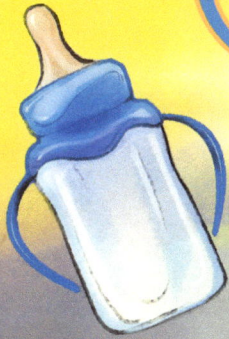

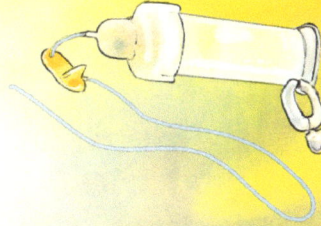

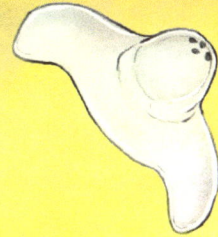

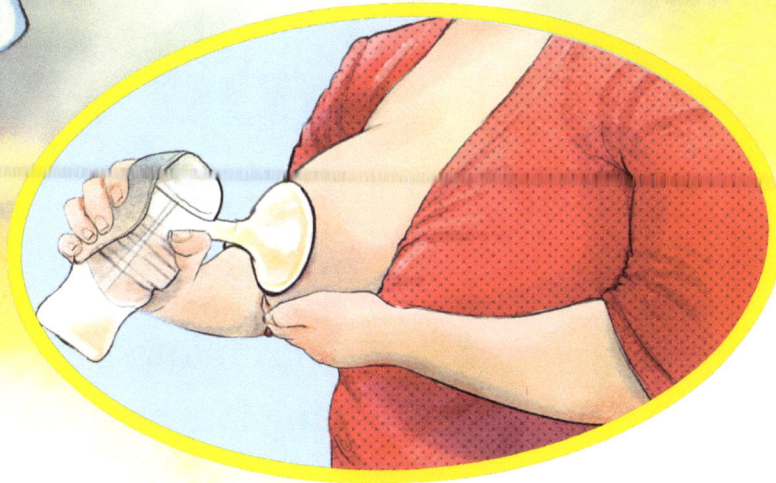

Every breastfeeding journey looks different. All are different lengths. Some journeys are only breast pumping. They can include a variety of devices and tools to make breastfeeding successful.

K

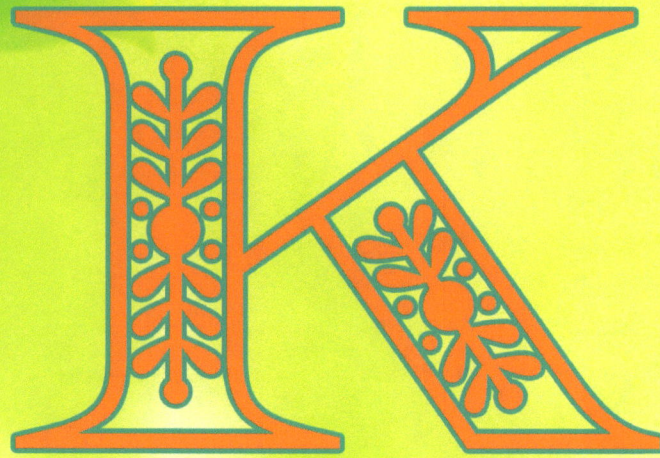

Kangaroo care
Kudos

Kangaroo care is an important step in the breastfeeding journey. It is when mother holds baby skin to skin. It helps to improve breast milk supply. Every mom that breastfeeds for any length of time deserves kudos, or praise.

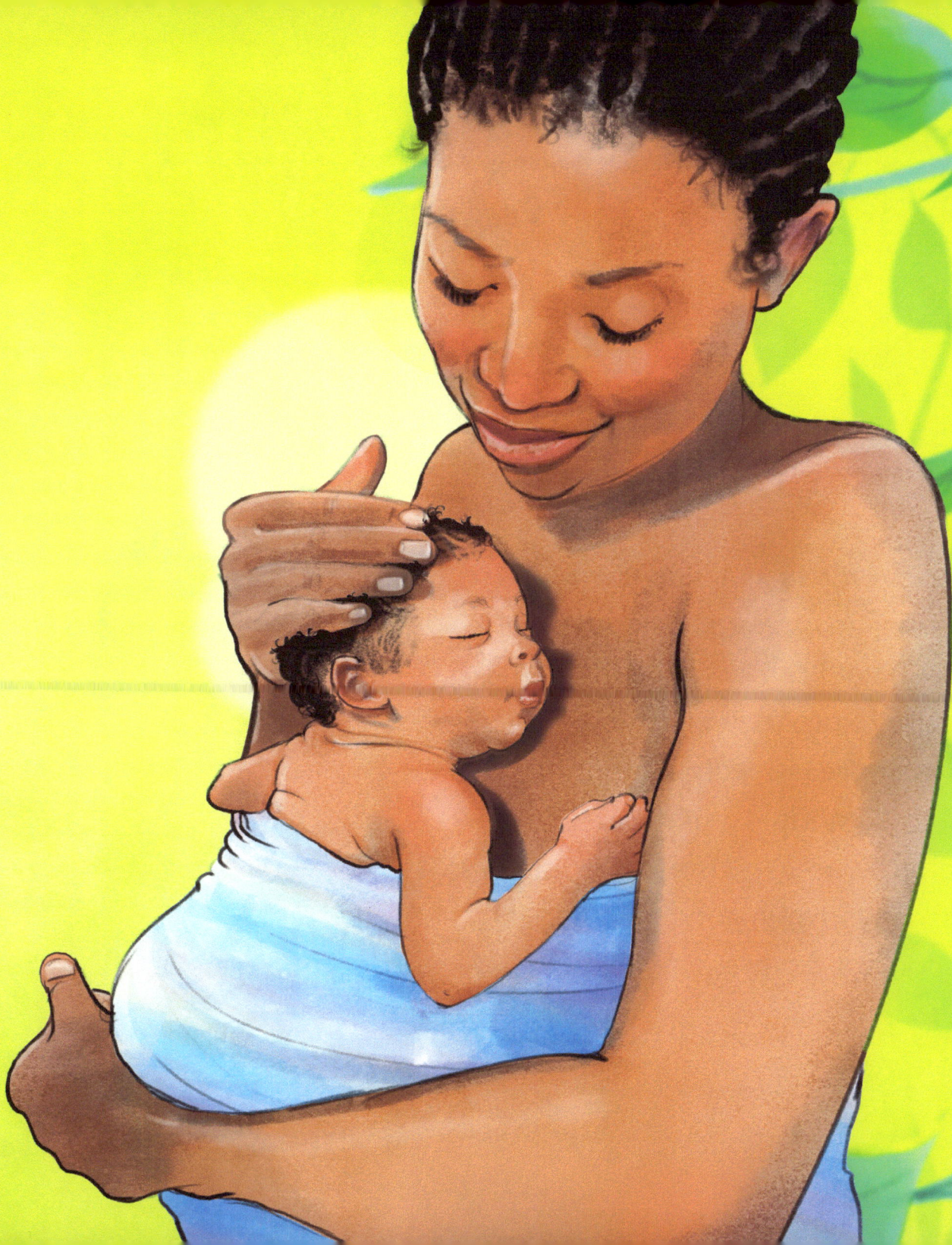

L

Liquid gold
Leak
Love
Latch

Breast milk is also known as liquid gold. A magical liquid gold! Liquid gold refers to the nutrient-rich milk produced in the early days of breastfeeding and its color. Sometimes milk can leak from the breasts. Breastfeeding provides love. A good latch is important for breastfeeding success.

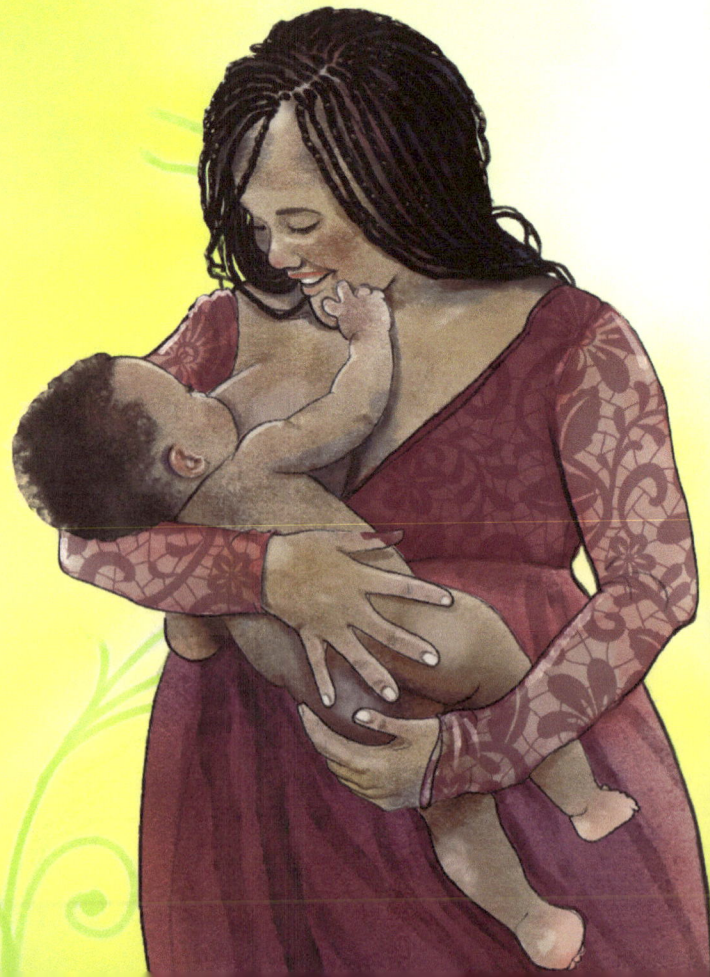

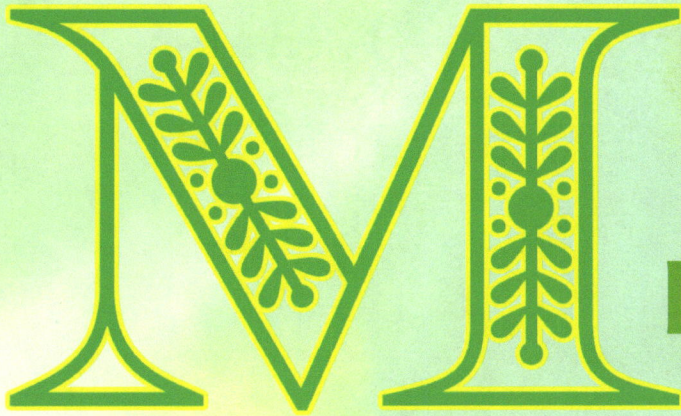

M Mouth Massage

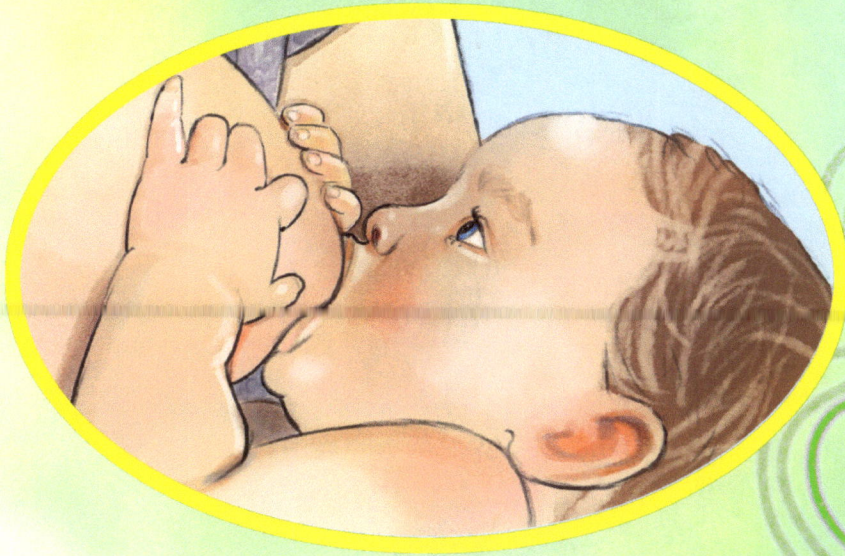

The **mouth** is an important body part in breastfeeding. Babies use their mouths to express milk. **Massaging** the breasts helps to express milk.

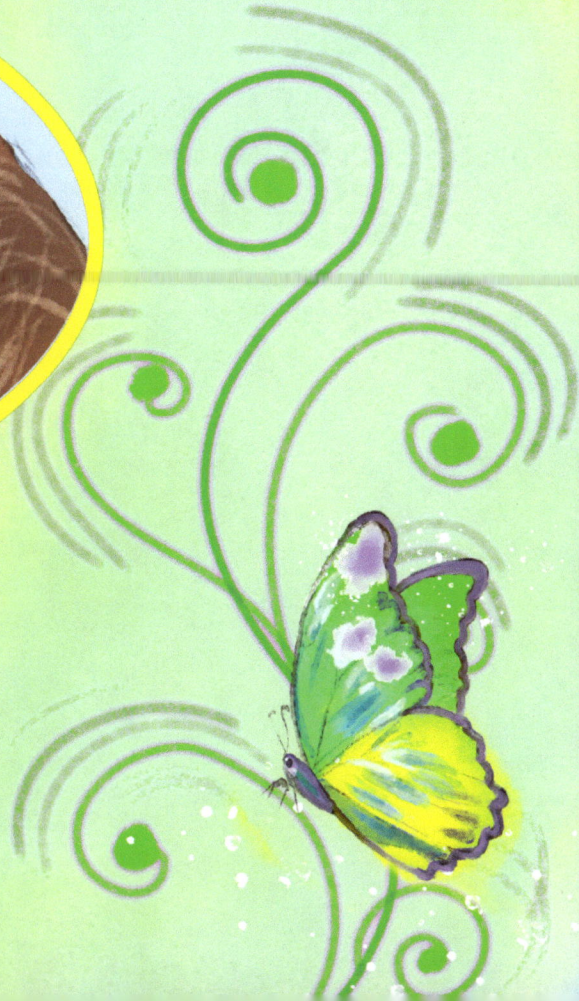

N

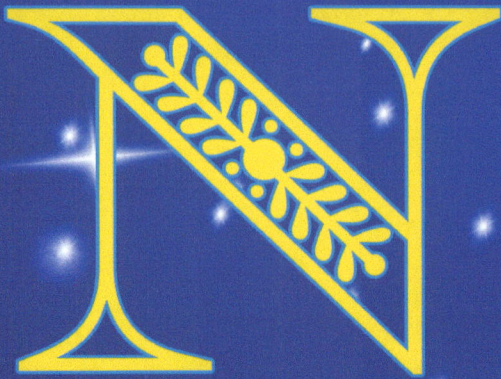

Nutrients
Natural
Night

Breastfeeding is a part of nature and provides many nutrients. It is natural for babies to wake to eat throughout the night.

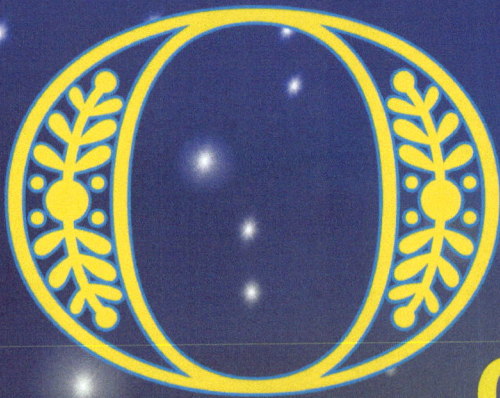

O

Breast milk is organic. It is a living milk. It contains cells and healthy bacteria. Oops! Sometimes moms or their helpers spill breast milk. Sometimes moms want to cry about the spilled milk.

Organic
Oops

P

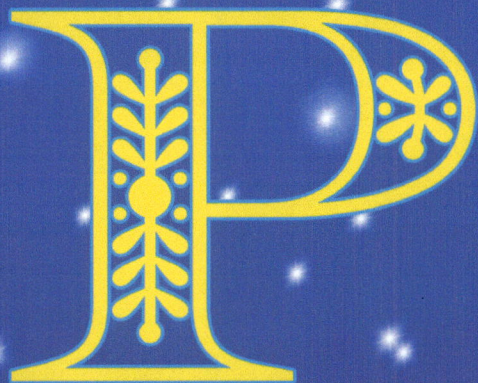

Pacify
Pump
Pillows
Public

Breastfeeding can help to **pacify**, or calm, baby. The breast **pump** can be used during the breastfeeding journey to express milk from breasts. **Pillows** can be used to achieve comfortable breastfeeding positions. Breastfeeding in **public** is allowed.

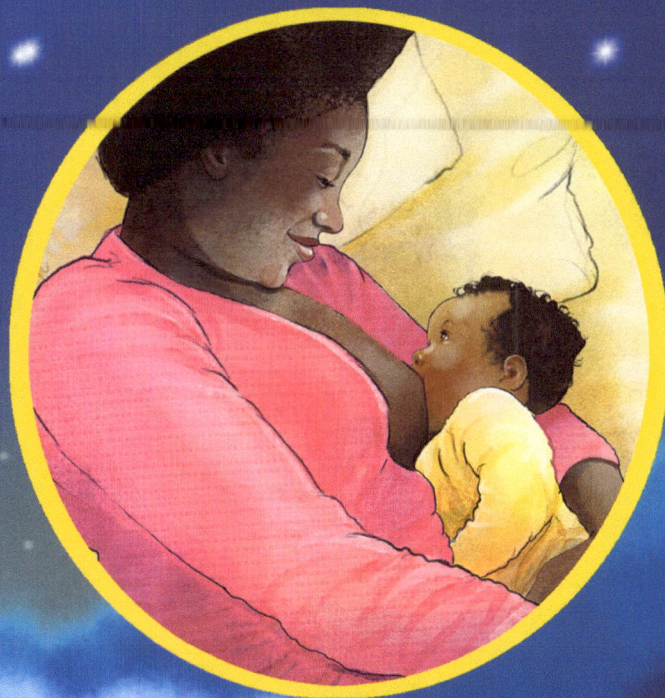

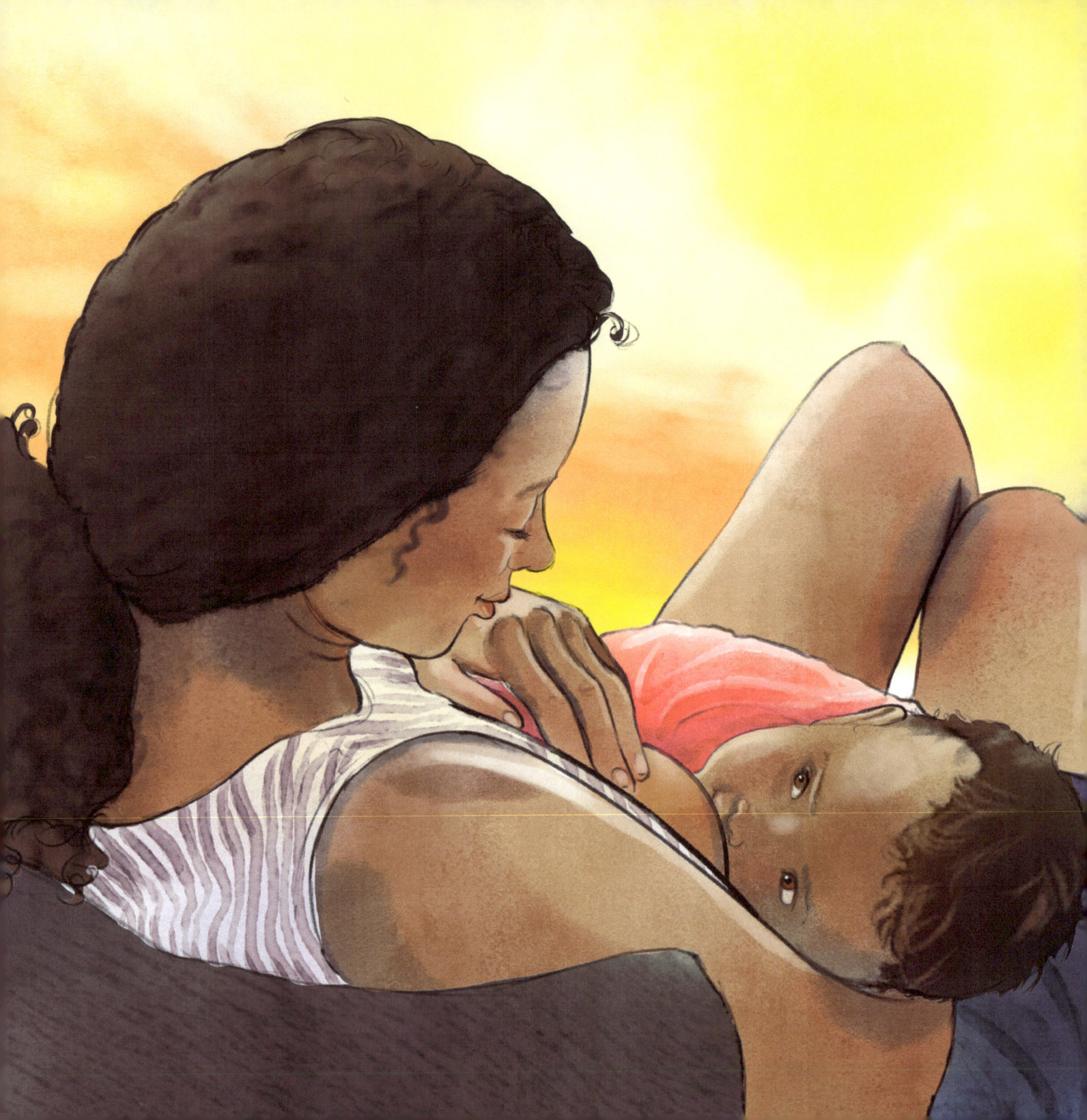

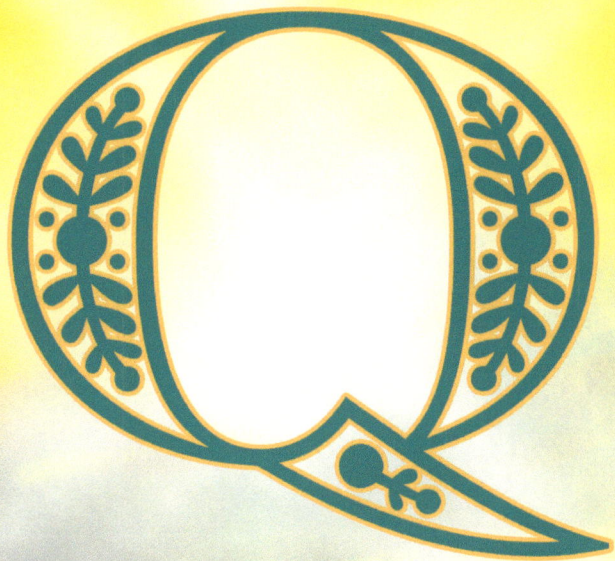

Quality time

Breastfeeding can be a time for mom and baby to spend quality time together.

Relax

Breastfeeding is a time when mom and baby can **relax** together.

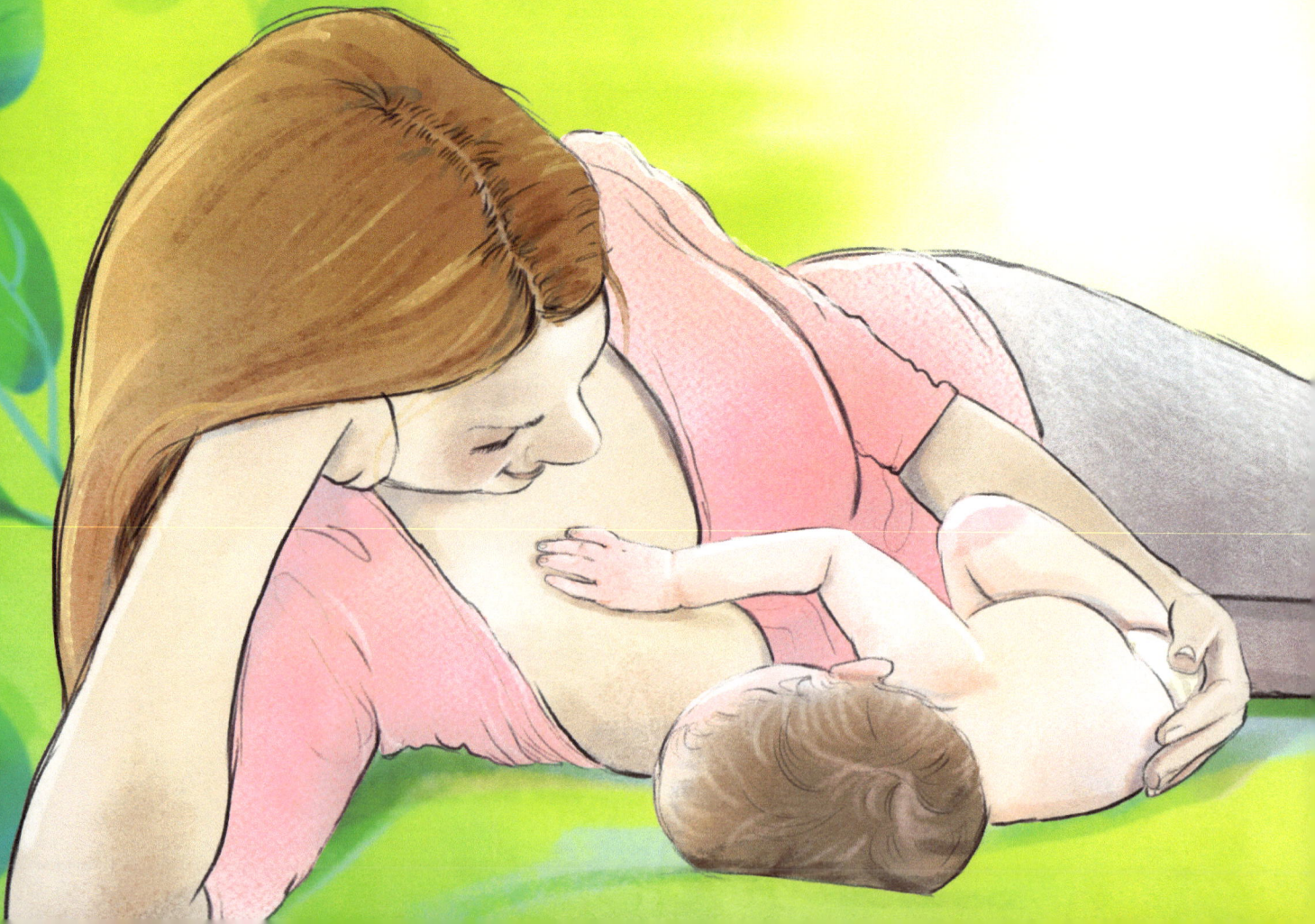

S

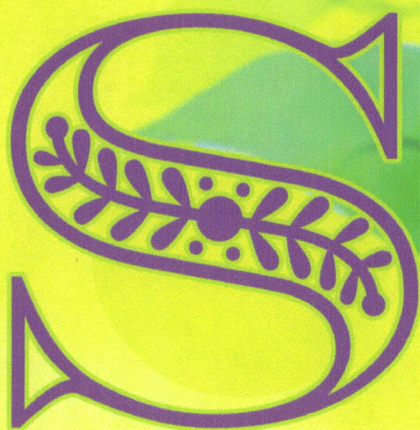

Suckle
Safety

To **suckle** is to feed by sucking at the breasts. Breastfeeding provides baby with a sense of **safety**.

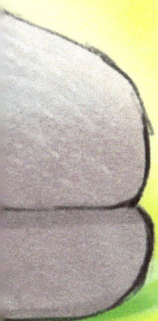

T

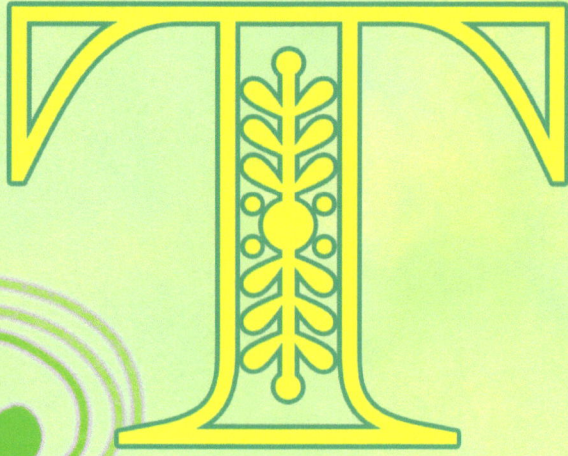

Tandem
Trust
Taste

Tandem feeding involves breastfeeding babies or children of two different ages at the same time. Breastfeeding builds trust between mother and baby. Breastfeeding involves mother trusting her body to do what it was designed to do. The taste of breast milk can change.

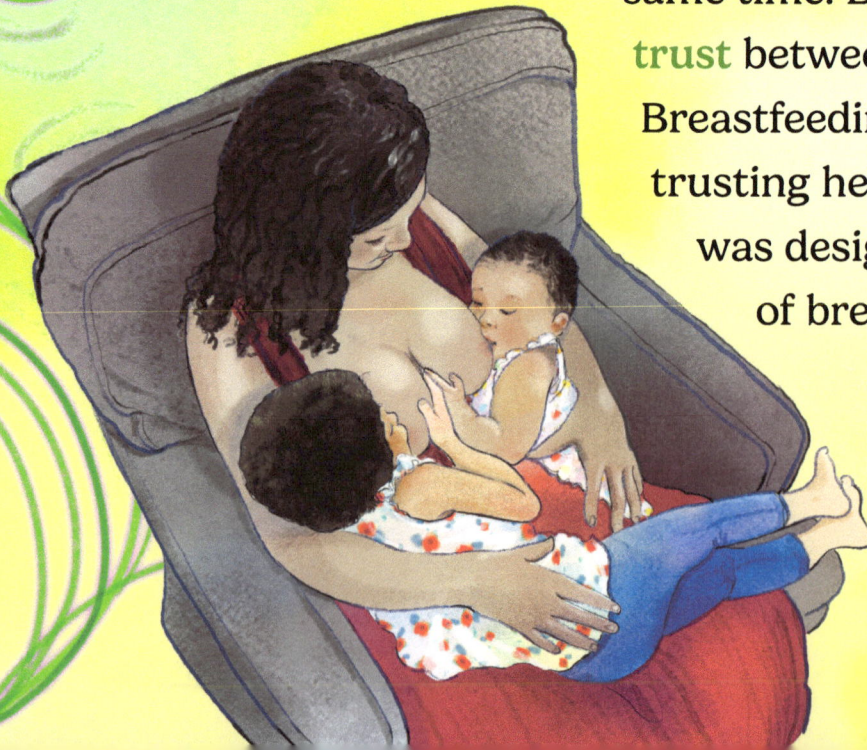

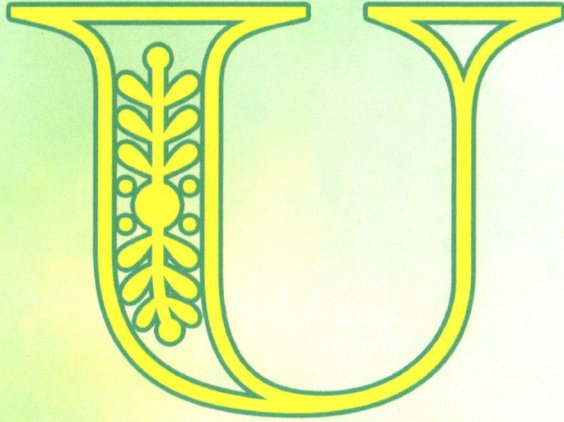

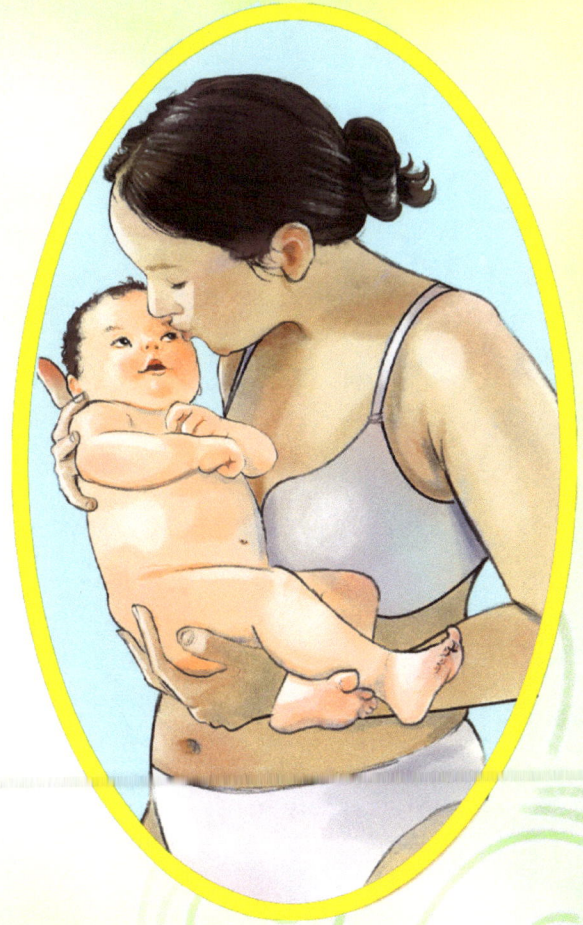

U

Unique

Every mother's breast milk is different. Breast milk changes to the needs of the baby. Every breastfeeding journey is unique.

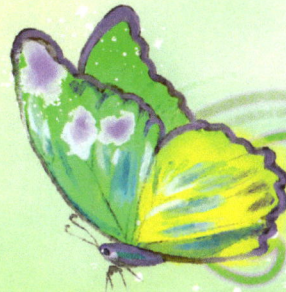

V

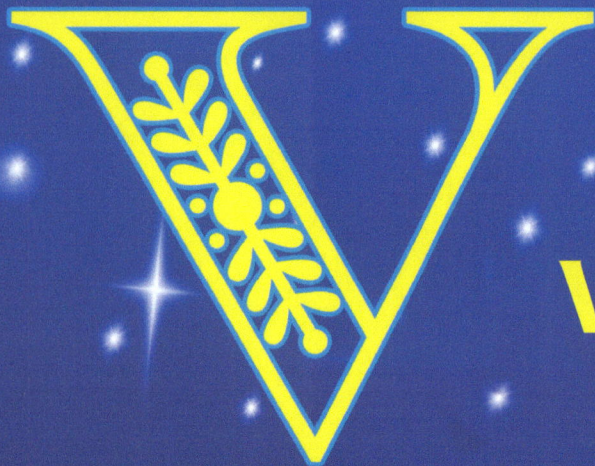

Village Vitamins

It takes a **village**, or many helpers, to create a successful breastfeeding journey. The breastfeeding journey is more successful when mom has the support of her partner, her family, and the community. Breast milk is healthy and provides important **vitamins**.

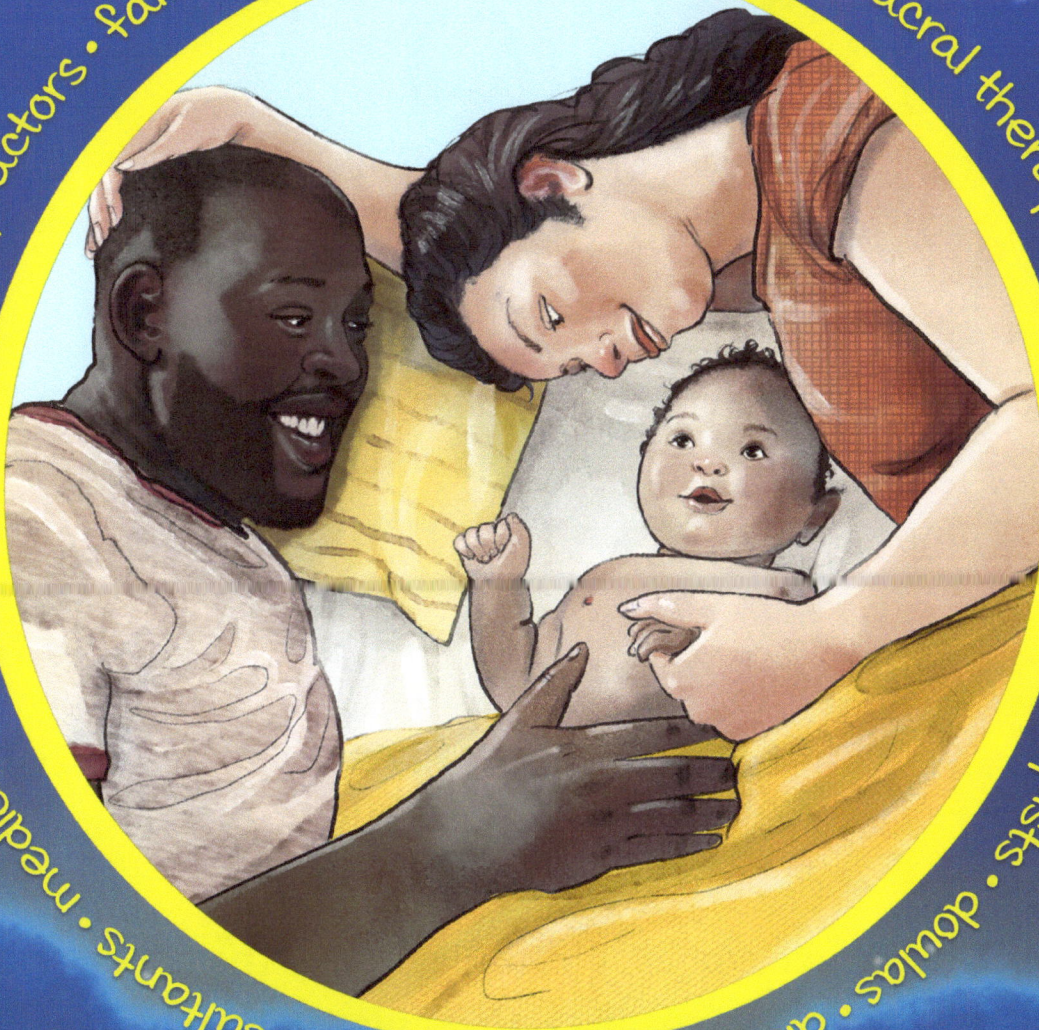

chiropractors • family • friends • midwives • craniosacral therapists • occupational therapists • doulas • dietitians • lactation consultants • medical doctors • nurses •

W

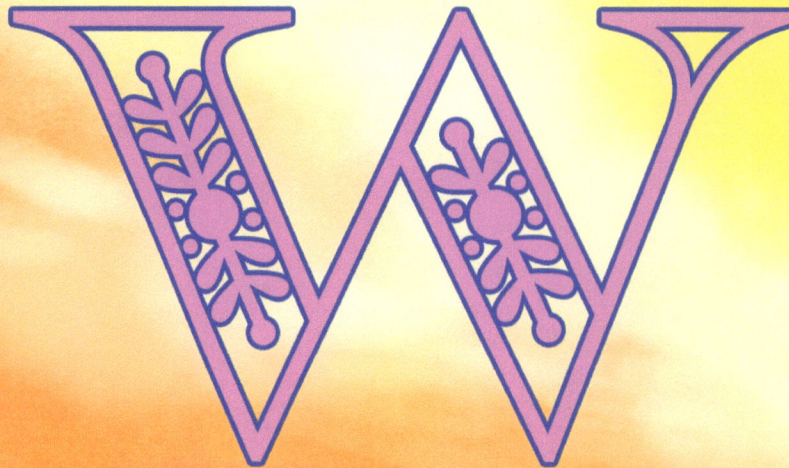

White
Wean
Work

Breast milk can be white. Eventually the dyad will wean, and the breastfeeding will come to an end. Moms can work and breastfeed.

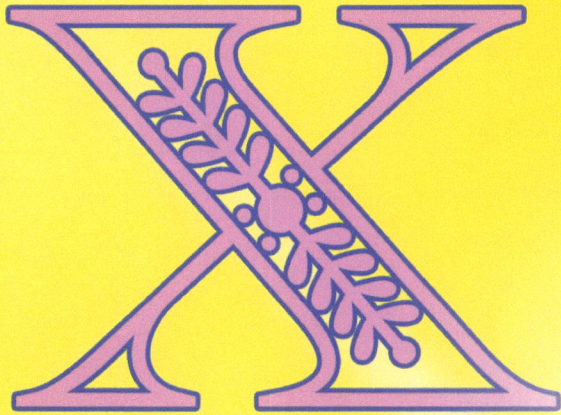

X

XO

Breastfeeding is a time to give baby hugs and kisses, or XOs.

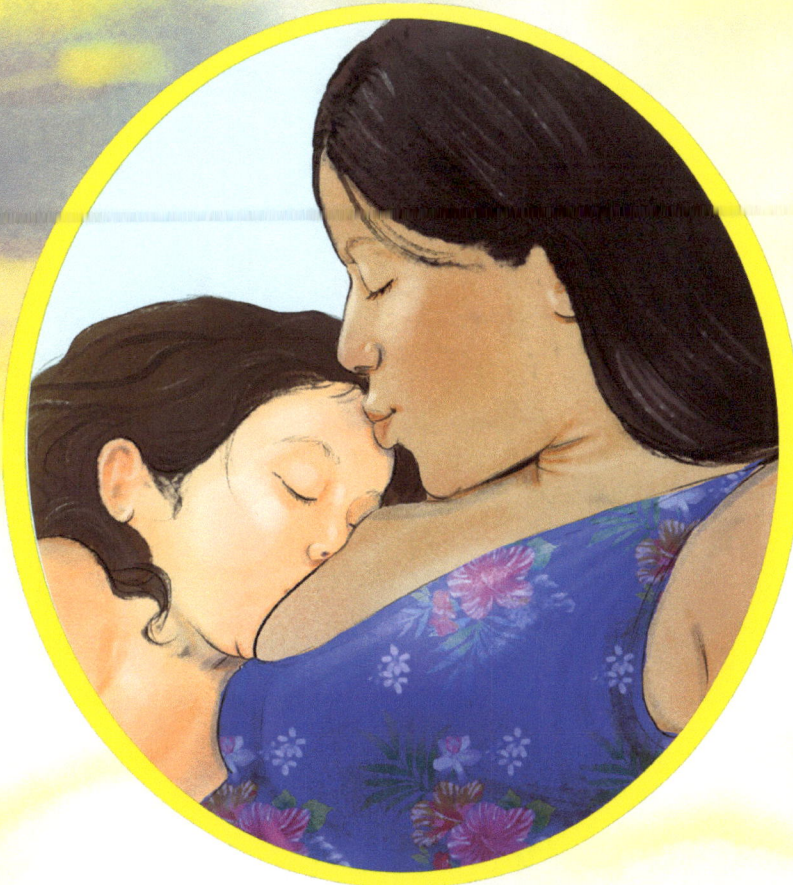

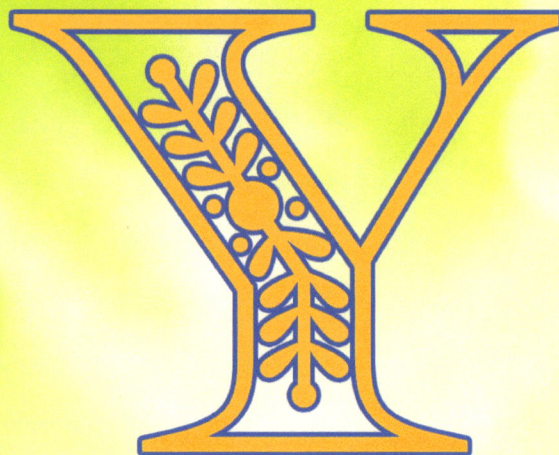

Y

Yellow
Yummy

Breast milk can be yellow.
Breast milk tastes yummy
to baby.

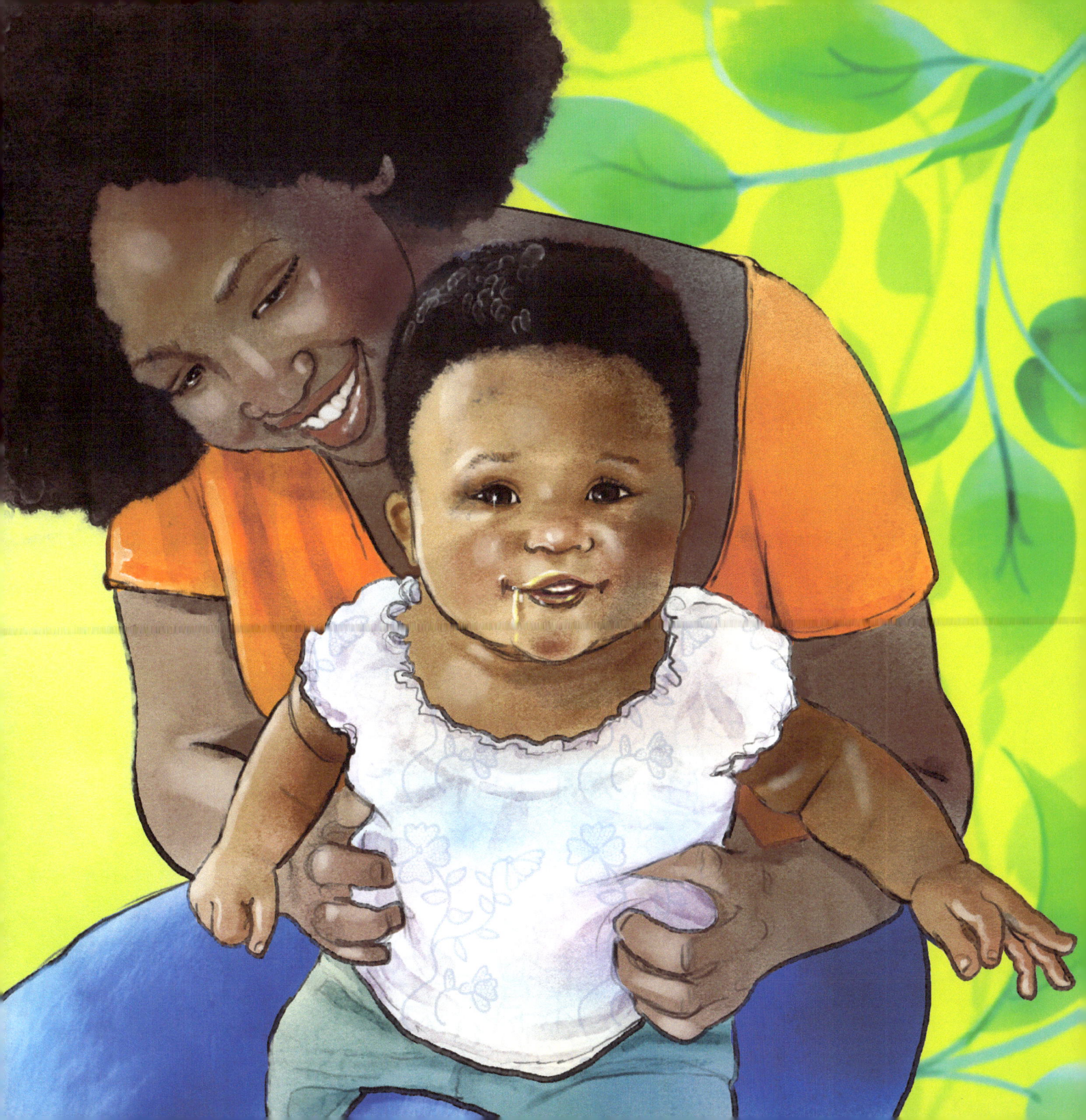

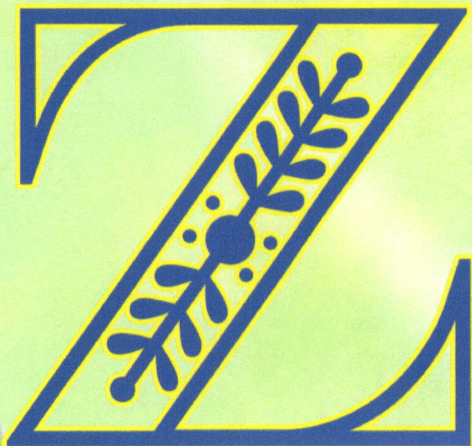

Z

Zzz

It is normal for babies to breastfeed themselves to sleep. Zzz.

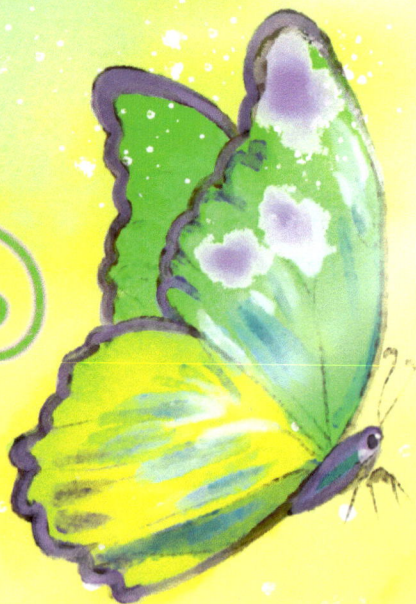

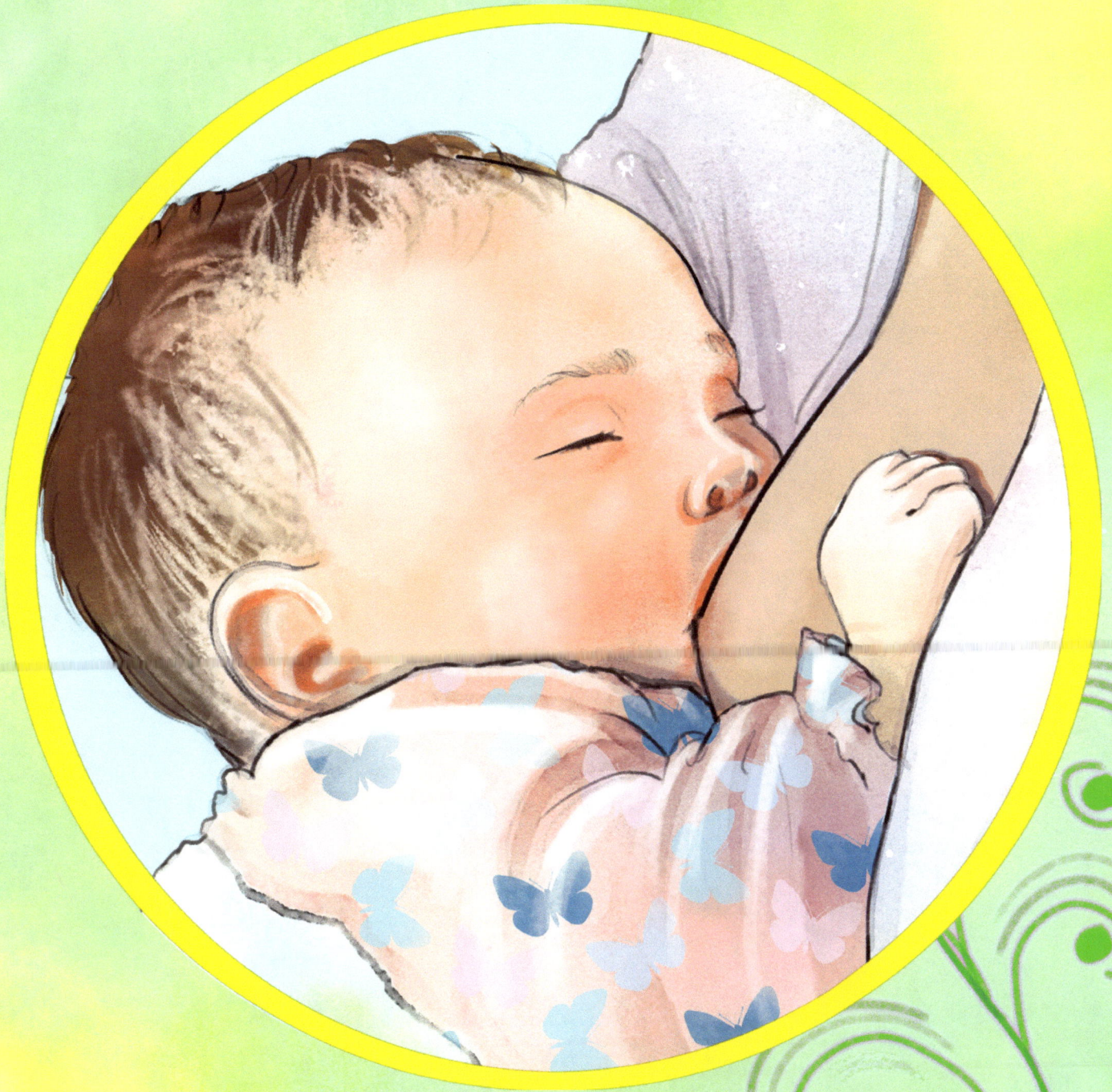

Now you know your
ABCs, won't you
support breastfeeding
with me?

www.ingramcontent.com/pod-product-compliance
Lightning Source LLC
Chambersburg PA
CBHW061144030426

42335CB00002B/95